ENDOMORPH DIET

STRATEGIC MEANS OF FOLLOWING THE
ENDOMORPH DIET

B. DANIELS

Contents

INTRODUCTION

Of the three main body types, endomorphs are characterized by an inherently high percentage of body fat and a propensity to gain weight quickly. The Endomorph Diet is intended for those with this body type in order to increase metabolism, regulate weight, and enhance overall health.

The key concepts often revolve around eating a balanced diet that prioritizes lean proteins, healthy fats, and complex carbohydrates. Nutrient-dense foods are prioritized to fulfill your hunger and provide essential vitamins and minerals; portion control is crucial.

Exercise is another crucial component; to enhance muscle mass and metabolism, strength training and cardiovascular workouts are prioritized. Achieving the right balance for your lifestyle and body type is essential.

Naturally, there are individual variations, so it's wise to seek particular advice from a dietitian or fitness professional. Do you have what it takes to be an endomorph?

CHAPTER ONE

The Summary of the Endomorph Body Type

The endomorph body type is one of the three somatotypes that characterize individuals based on their underlying physical traits and tendency to acquire or lose weight. The following is a summary of the endomorph:

Physical characteristics:

Increase in Body Fat: Endomorphs typically have a higher percentage of body fat, which promotes weight growth.

Rounder Shape: Their bodies are often soft and rounded, with fat stored in the thighs, hips, and stomach.

The rate of metabolism

Slower Metabolism: Endomorphs' slower metabolic rates may make them less efficient calorie burners.

Muscle Mass:

Naturally Strong: Endomorphs usually have a stronger, more robust body type.

Potential for Muscle grow: They could not only need to effectively grow muscle but also manage fat accumulation.

Problems

Handling Weight: Endomorphs may find it more difficult to lose weight, therefore they should use caution when choosing their diet and exercise routine.

Fat Storage: Because excess calories are frequently stored as fat, following a well-planned diet is essential.

Nutritional Requirements:

Balanced Diet: Eating meals rich in nutrients and minimizing portion sizes are key components of the Endomorph Diet, which aims to achieve a balanced intake of macronutrients.

Activities to Try:

Together: It's often recommended to follow a well-rounded fitness routine that incorporates both strength training and aerobic activities to boost metabolism and help with weight management.

It's crucial to keep in mind that, although somatotypes provide a general framework, individuals may combine characteristics from several body types. Nutrition and exercise regimens must be tailored to the individual needs and preferences of each person in order to promote and maintain a healthy lifestyle.

The significance of modifying nutrition according to body type

It can be beneficial to customize your diet to your body type for a number of reasons. The rationale behind tailoring your diet to your specific requirements is as follows:

Optimal Nutritional Intake:

The amount of nutrients that different body types require can vary. You can ensure that your body is getting the right amount of macronutrients (proteins, fats, and carbohydrates) and micronutrients (vitamins and minerals) for optimal function by tailoring your diet.

Handling Your Weight:

Your understanding of your body type may help you better understand how different meals affect your body. Understanding this information will enable you to make more informed decisions to better manage your weight, regardless of your objectives weight reduction, maintenance, or growth.

Energy Degrees:

The right balance of foods might affect your energy levels. You may prevent energy slumps and fatigue by tailoring your diet to provide your body with the nourishment it requires for sustained energy levels all day.

Developing and Preserving Muscle:

Customizing your diet to fit your body type can help you gain and keep muscle. Those who engage in strength training or other physical activities should pay particular attention to this.

Aid to the Metabolic Process:

Variations exist in the metabolic rates of several body types. By adjusting your food, you can boost your metabolism and achieve your goals of losing weight or ensuring that your endomorph body type is utilizing its energy reserves.

Digestive Health:

Some individuals may have sensitivities or preferences about their digestive systems. You may enhance your overall health and gut health by customizing your diet to include items that work well for your digestive system.

Adherence and Long-Term Success:

A diet that suits your preferences and body type will probably be more maintainable in the long run. This increases compliance and generally assists you in reaching your nutritional goals.

While considering your body type is vital, it's also important to recognize personal preferences and variances. Consult a nutritionist or other healthcare professional for personalized guidance based on your unique needs. This will guarantee that the foods you select will help you reach your fitness and general health goals.

Being aware of endomorphs

DNA Predisposition:

Endomorphs are genetically predisposed to gaining fat more readily than those with other body types. This is often attributed to slower metabolism and higher body fat percentages.

Makeup for the Body:

Usually with a softer, rounder frame, they have more body fat, especially in the thighs, hips, and abdomen.

Potential for Muscle Growth:

Despite their propensity to accumulate fat, endomorphs typically have a solid foundation for muscle growth. If they follow the right diet and training regimen, they can grow a strong, muscular physique.

Endomorphs may experience difficulties with a reduced rate of metabolism, which lowers their pace of burning calories. Despite this, controlling weight is still doable even though it can be a bit more challenging at times.

Difficulties with Weight Loss:

They could struggle to lose weight in comparison to people with different body types. However, if diet and exercise are done correctly, significant and long-lasting weight loss is attainable.

The Endomorph Diet often emphasizes portion management and maintaining a balance of macronutrients. Lean proteins, healthy fats, and complex carbohydrates all significantly support their goals.

Activities to Try:

A comprehensive fitness program for endomorphs should include both cardiovascular exercises, which boost metabolism and burn calories, and strength training, which develops muscle and can increase resting metabolic rate.

CHAPTER TWO

Adaptability

Although endomorphs possess some attributes, they can also possess characteristics of other body types. It is imperative that food and fitness be approached individually, taking into consideration personal preferences and variances.

You may learn a lot about how your body responds to different stimuli by understanding your body type, whether it be endomorph or any other somatotype. It gives you the structure to successfully reach your fitness and health goals by modifying your diet, exercise routine, and way of life. Remember that rather than placing constraints on yourself, developing a sustainable and healthy lifestyle requires working with your body.

Dietary Guidelines for Endomorphs

Let us look at some key dietary recommendations that are special to endomorphs:

Balanced Macronutrients:

Ensure that the three macronutrients—fats, proteins, and carbohydrates—that you eat are all in balance. Try to eat lean protein, healthy fats, and carbohydrates in moderation for the sake of your overall health.

Managed Amount:

Because fat accumulates fat more easily, portions need to be regulated. Consider portion proportions in order to limit your intake of calories and prevent overindulging.

Sophisticated Carbs:

Choose lower-GI foods like whole grains, vegetables, and legumes for your complex carbohydrate intake. They provide sustained energy and aid in blood sugar regulation.

Slim-Joining Proteins:

Lean protein sources can aid in the development and maintenance of muscle. Opt for fish, chicken, tofu, lentils, and low-fat dairy products.

Good fats

Incorporate foods high in unsaturated fats, such as avocados, nuts, seeds, and olive oil. These fats not only improve your overall health but also have the ability to fill you up.

Foods High in Fibre:

You can increase your fiber intake by eating more fruits, vegetables, and whole grains. Fiber promotes healthy digestion, helps control appetite, and may even help with weight management.

Frequently Eaten & Snack:

Aim for frequent, well-balanced meals to maintain steady energy levels throughout the day. Eat wholesome snacks in between meals to curb hunger and prevent overindulging.

Drinking enough water

To stay hydrated during the day, sip on plenty of water. Water is essential for several bodily functions, including weight management, and it makes you feel fuller for longer.

Limit foods with added sugar and processed foods:

Limit the quantity of processed and sugar-added foods that you eat. These might not provide the necessary nutrients, which could result in overindulging in calories.

When Meals Are Taken:

Consider your eating schedule. Eat a balanced diet, for instance, both before and after working out. This can support overall fitness goals, muscle recovery, and energy levels.

Regular Exercise Routine:

Meals are just a part of the overall. A balanced diet and regular exercise that incorporates both strength training and aerobic activity can help with weight management and boost metabolism.

Remember at all times that although these rules provide a broad base, individual tastes and differences should be taken into account. A nutritionist or other healthcare professional can help you establish a personalized food plan that

meets your specific needs and goals as an
endomorph.

To support their goals for health and fitness,
endomorphs would like to prioritize the
following types of foods in their diets:

Sophisticated Carbs:

Good options for snacks include sweet potatoes,
quinoa, brown rice, and oats. They have less of
an impact on blood sugar levels, are rich in fiber,
and provide consistent energy.

Slim-Joining Proteins:

Fish, turkey, chicken breast, lentils, tofu, and low-fat dairy are examples of foods high in lean protein. Protein is essential for muscular growth and might make you feel fuller.

Good fats

Add sources of healthy fats such as avocados, nuts, seeds, and olive oil. These fats contribute to satiety in addition to providing essential nutrients.

Produce and Fruits:

Stock up on a variety of colorful fruits and vegetables. They are rich in antioxidants, vitamins, and minerals and low in calories.

Low-Carb Cheeses and Cheese Alternatives:

Add low-fat or fat-free dairy products, or dairy alternatives such soy or almond milk. They provide essential calcium and protein.

High-Protein Snacks:

Have a snack of high-protein food, like almonds, Greek yogurt, or cottage cheese. High-protein snacks can help reduce hunger in between meals.

Items High in Fibre:

Increase your intake of high-fiber foods such as vegetables, beans, lentils, and whole grains. Fiber promotes a healthy digestive system and helps control hunger.

Drinks to Help Rehydrate:

You can stay hydrated by drinking water and herbal teas. It's crucial for your general health and might make you feel fuller if you drink enough water.

Green tea:

Green tea's constituents may quicken your metabolism. Make it a part of your routine as a calorie-free beverage option.

Nutrition Before and After Physical Activity:

Prioritize eating a well-balanced meal before and after your activity that includes both protein and carbohydrates. This helps with energy levels, muscle growth, and overall fitness goals.

Portion sizes on average:

Consider the proportions of your portions to avoid overindulging. Use smaller plates, be aware of when your body is hungry or full, and savor your meal.

Remember that these are only general suggestions and that nutritional needs and preferences may vary. To create a long-lasting, personalized eating plan that suits your specific requirements as an endomorph, you should always seek advice from a nutritionist or other medical practitioner.

Things You Should Limit or Avoid

Endomorphs should limit their intake of or avoid the following foods:

Product of processing: food

Reduce your intake of highly processed foods since they usually contain extra sugars, unhealthy fats, and preservatives. Overindulging in calories could be attributed to these.

Dessert Drinks:

Avoid sodas, energy drinks, and fruit juices that have been sweetened. It's preferable to stick to water or other low-calorie beverages like herbal teas.

Richly Manipulated Carbohydrates:

Eat fewer refined carbohydrates, which are included in white bread, sugary cereals, and pastries. Blood sugar levels may spike as a result of these.

High-Sugar Snacks:

Cut back on the candies, pastries, and high-sugar snacks you eat. Choose healthier alternatives, such as fruit or nuts, when you have a sweet tooth.

High-fat or fried foods:

Eat less items that are really greasy and fried. Use cooking methods that are healthy, such baking, grilling, or steaming.

Excessive Use of Dairy Fat:

Reduce your intake of high-fat dairy products. Select low-fat or fat-free goods to reduce overall calorie and saturated fat consumption.

Alcoholic Drink:

Moderate alcohol consumption is advised since it might contribute to an excessive calorie intake and possibly make it more difficult to lose weight.

Meats that have been prepared:

Eat less processed meats, such as hot dogs, sausages, and bacon, as they might be high in unhealthy fats and sodium.

Overconsumption of Sugar and Pastries:

Limit the quantity of sweets, pastries, and baked goods you eat. These often include processed carbs and unhealthy fats.

Snacks High in Energy:

Be cautious while consuming high-calorie snacks, particularly if they don't include many nutrients. Opt for snacks that are high in nutrients, including fruits, vegetables, or high-protein foods.

Sugar-Added Condiments and Sauces:

Check sauce and condiment labels for added sugars. Select handmade or carefully chosen goods that have minimal or no added sugar.

Never forget that moderation is the key to finding a long-lasting balance that works for your particular tastes and style of living. It's always a good idea to consult a nutritionist or other healthcare provider to create a personalized food plan that fits your specific requirements as an endomorph.

When and How Much Food Should Be Eaten

When and how often endomorphs eat are crucial factors in achieving their fitness and health goals. Remember the following when deciding when and how often to eat:

Regular Meals:

Eat consistent, well-balanced meals throughout the day. Meal timing helps control blood sugar levels and provides a steady source of energy.

Eat Three Main Meals and Snacks:

Consider having three main meals a day: dinner, lunch, and breakfast. Snackle on healthy foods in between meals. This tactic can help you prevent overindulging during main meals and maintain steady energy levels.

Diet Prior to Exercise:

Eat a healthy meal that consists of a mix of carbohydrates and protein before working exercise. This sustains vitality and provides the energy required for physical activity.

Nutrition following a workout:

Consume a high-protein, high-carbohydrate lunch or snack after your workout. This encourages muscle regeneration and replenishes glycogen storage.

A Balanced Breakfast:

To increase your metabolism and give you energy for the entire morning, make sure your breakfast is nutritious and well-balanced.

Responsible Consumption:

Recognize when you are hungry and full. Eat whenever you feel like it to avoid overindulging, but try not to wait until you're really hungry.

Prevent Heavy, Late-Night Eats:

Nearer to nighttime, eat lighter meals. Opt for a lighter dinner to facilitate better digestion and prevent pain during sleep.

The Appropriate Time to Hydrate:

Throughout the day, stay hydrated, but avoid drenching yourself with water shortly before or right after meals to prevent your digestive enzymes from becoming diluted. For improved digestion, sip water between meals.

Dependable Time

Strive to follow a consistent daily routine for meals and snacks. This helps to keep your metabolism healthy overall by controlling your body's internal clock.

Be mindful of your body:

Keep track of how your body responds to different meal timings and quantities. Modifications can be necessary based on lifestyle choices and personal preferences.

Keep from skipping meals:

Avoid missing meals since this might affect metabolism and lead to overindulgence in the later part of the day. Frequent meal and snack consumption helps control energy levels.

It's critical to choose meal times and intervals that fit your lifestyle, bearing in mind that everyone has different tastes and timetables. You can get advice specifically tailored to your needs as an endomorph by speaking with a dietitian or other medical professional.

Water consumption

Regardless of body type, it's critical for everyone to drink enough water, but endomorph diet goals require it even more. Endomorphs should take the following into account when it comes to hydration:

Water Use:

To stay adequately hydrated during the day, make sure you consume enough water. Water is essential for several biological activities, including digestion, absorption of nutrients, and metabolism.

The Right Time to Drink Water:

Drink water regularly throughout the day. Try not to wait until you're really thirsty because sometimes thirst might be mistaken for appetite.

CHAPTER THREE

Between meals, sip water:

Even though being hydrated is crucial, try not to consume a lot of water during meals. Drinking too much water right before or after meals may dilute digestive enzymes and make digestion harder.

Drink plenty of water before and after working out.

Prioritize staying hydrated prior to, during, and following physical activity. For optimal athletic performance, muscle function, and recovery, enough hydration is crucial.

Meals with a High Water Content:

Include items that are high in water in your diet, such fruits and vegetables. These promote both hydration and nutrient consumption.

Monitor Liquid Loss:

Be mindful of circumstances such as intense physical exertion, high temperatures, or certain medications that may elevate the risk of fluid loss. Adapt how much water you drink to the circumstances.

Reduce Sugar- and Calorie-Rich Drinks:

Restrict your use of sugar-filled, high-calorie drinks as they may cause you to overindulge in calories. Avoid sugar-filled beverages and stick to water or herbal teas.

Drinking Enough Water and Managing Your Weight:

Drinking adequate water can aid with weight management by promoting satiety. Occasionally, the body may confuse thirst for hunger.

The Various Hydration Needs of Each Person:

Everybody has different needs when it comes to hydration, so listen to your body. Depending on your age, activity level, and surroundings, your water needs can change.

Hydration and Energy Production:

optimal hydration is related to an optimal metabolism. Consistently drinking water should be your first priority because even a small amount of dehydration might impact metabolic efficiency.

Remember that the "8x8 rule" eight 8-ounce glasses of water each day is merely a general suggestion and that each person has varied water requirements. Adjust your water consumption based on your lifestyle and particular needs. If you have any specific health concerns or conditions, it's always a good idea to consult a healthcare professional for personalized advice on hydration.

Exercise and Movement

Physical activity and exercise are essential components of an endomorph's quest to support their fitness and health goals. Exercise gives the following benefits in addition to the endomorph diet:

Combining Exercise for Cardiovascular and Strength:

Include both strength training and aerobic activities such as swimming, cycling, or running in your workout routine to ensure it is well-rounded. While strength training builds muscle mass and accelerates the burning of calories, cardio exercise raises the resting metabolic rate.

Increasing Your Stomach:

Endomorphs, who may naturally have a slower metabolism, can benefit from frequent exercise to help speed up their metabolism. This might support weight control and fat loss.

Using Up Calories:

Exercise boosts caloric expenditure, which results in an energy deficit that supports weight loss. A balanced diet and regular exercise are necessary to achieve and maintain a healthy weight.

Training in intervals:

Consider incorporating interval training into your cardiovascular workouts. High-intensity intervals have the potential to improve cardiovascular fitness and increase fat burning.

Strength Training for Muscle Building:

Strength training is crucial for endomorphs to maintain and develop muscle mass. Muscle tissue increases calorie expenditure while at rest, supporting a normal metabolism in general.

Continuous Timetable:

Maintaining consistency is the key. Make an effort to adhere to a consistent training plan that rotates between strength and cardio workouts each week.

Nutrition following a workout:

Following a workout, consider your diet. Eating a balanced breakfast or snack that contains both protein and carbohydrates will help replenish glycogen levels after exercise and promote muscle regeneration.

Observe Preferences:

Choose activities you enjoy doing to make fitness sustainable. Finding activities you enjoy doing increases the likelihood that you will stick to your fitness routine, whether it be dancing, hiking, or weightlifting.

Being Aware of Motion:

Allocate more time in your daily schedule for physical activities. Elevate your physical activity level with simple exercises like stretching, walking, and using the stairs.

Drinking enough water

Make sure you stay hydrated before, during, and after any physical exercise. Adequate water helps in recovery and overall performance.

Consult a Fitness Professional for Advice:

When in doubt, consult a fitness expert or personal trainer to make sure your workout regimen is customized to your objectives, degree of fitness, and any potential restrictions. Regular exercise along with a balanced diet is the key to achieving and maintaining a healthy lifestyle. To prevent injury and overtraining, customize your workout to your preferences and always pay attention to your body.

Additionals for Endomorphs

While some supplements can support overall health and fitness goals and work well with an endomorph diet, most nutrients are better received from whole foods. The following supplements might be something endomorphs want to consider:

Powdered Protein:

If endomorphs struggle to receive enough protein from whole meals, using protein powder as a supplement may help them meet their needs. Pick premium protein powders such as casein, whey, or pea.

Omega-three fish oils:

Fish oil or algal oil capsules are examples of omega-3 supplements that include essential fatty acids that support heart health and reduce inflammation.

Several nutrients:

A multivitamin can help close any potential dietary nutrient deficits by ensuring that the body receives enough of the essential vitamins and minerals.

Vitamin D:

Low vitamin D levels can affect people of all body kinds, particularly those who don't get enough sun exposure. The immune system and bones can benefit from extra vitamin D.

Calcium:

Endomorphs, like everyone else, need adequate calcium for strong bones. If you're not eating enough, you can benefit from taking a calcium supplement.

Supplements containing fiber:

If it's hard to acquire enough fiber from natural meals, a fiber supplement might aid in digestion and encourage fullness.

Supplements for your Warm-Up:

Some endomorphs who want to boost their energy and focus before working out may find pre-workout medications useful. However, you should choose these carefully and consult a healthcare professional before using them.

BCAAs, or branch-chain amino acids:

BCAAs can help repair damaged muscles and reduce soreness after intense exercise. These are especially useful for individuals who practice strength training on a regular basis.

Antioxidants found in green tea extract may aid in metabolism. As a supplement, you can use it, but first make sure it helps you achieve your health goals.

CLA, or conjugated linoleic acid:

CLA supplements are supposed to help reduce body fat while preserving muscle mass. However, it's crucial to see a physician before utilizing this supplement due to the contradictory studies.

Remember that not every person needs supplements, and that a balanced diet should always come first. To ensure that supplements suit your goals, needs, and current health status, you should visit a trained dietitian or healthcare professional before adding any.

Adopting a comprehensive strategy for lifestyle and behavior changes can significantly improve the endomorph diet. The following are some significant behavioral and lifestyle changes to consider:

Responsible Consumption:

Become aware of your body's cues when it comes to hunger and fullness to practice mindful eating. Eat quietly and savor each bite of your meal.

Regular Movement:

Make sure to include both cardiovascular and strength training in your daily fitness regimen. Aim for at least 150 minutes per week of moderate-to-intense aerobic activity.

Obtaining Sufficient Sleep:

Make getting enough rest a top priority. The hormonal balance can be upset by sleep deprivation, which can affect hunger and metabolism. The aim is to get seven to nine hours of good sleep every night.

Stress Mitigation:

Take part in relaxing exercises like yoga, deep breathing, or meditation to relieve stress. Extended stress may impact metabolism and result in weight gain.

CHAPTER FOUR

Accept a community that exists to support you. Speak with loved ones who can encourage you and hold you responsible for achieving your fitness and wellness goals.

Making a Meal Plan:

Plan and prepare meals ahead of time to avoid impulsive or bad eating choices. Having healthful meals readily available will help sustain an endomorph diet.

Hydration Schedules:

Make it your routine to drink enough of water throughout the day. You can more easily meet your daily water intake goals if you always carry a water bottle.

Determining Goals:

Set realistic and reachable objectives for your diet and exercise. Divide more ambitious goals into more manageable milestones so that you can celebrate your accomplishments along the way.

Get Knowledgeable:

Learn more about healthy eating, exercise, and lifestyle choices. You may make decisions that are consistent with your goals when you possess knowledge.

When Meals Are Taken:

Make meal plans ahead of time to help keep blood sugar levels consistent and avoid becoming overly hungry, which can lead to overindulgence.

Self-Encouraging Reminder:

Have a positive attitude. Show off your progress rather than focusing on perfection. No matter how small, acknowledge and celebrate all of your successes, and practice self-compassion.

Behavior in Counseling:

Seek advice from a behavioral counselor or certified dietitian. They can provide you with customized ideas and support to help you transition to a sustainable lifestyle.

Observation Follow-Up:

Maintain a food and exercise diary to track your progress. This can help identify patterns, advantages, and areas that need improvement.

Remembering that long-term lifestyle changes call for perseverance and patience is crucial. Tailored to your own needs and tastes, these modifications can help you succeed on the endomorph diet over the long run.

Observing Changes and Advancements

All dietary and lifestyle adjustments, including the endomorph diet, need to be followed with careful observation of outcomes and appropriate modification. Here are some effective methods for keeping an eye on your progress and making the necessary adjustments:

Make sure your goals are clear:

Decide on specific, measurable, and reachable goals. Whether the objective is to gain more muscle, reduce weight, or enhance general health, having defined goals provides guidance.

Regular Assessments:

To track your progress, schedule frequent test-taking sessions. Measures, body weight, body fat percentage, and fitness evaluations may be part of this.

Keeping a Diary of Food:

Maintain a detailed food journal to track your daily caloric intake. This helps identify potential areas for improvement, assess the nutritional balance, and identify trends.

Activity Log:

Make a note of the type, duration, and intensity of each workout session in your fitness journal. This diary will allow you to monitor your improvement in terms of strength, endurance, and overall fitness.

Measurements and images:

Take measurements and progress photos on a regular basis. Changes in body composition may not always register immediately on the scale, despite the fact that images and measurements may provide you with a more comprehensive view of your progress.

Monitor Your Level of Energy:

Throughout the day, monitor your level of energy. An increase in energy could indicate that you're making good dietary and lifestyle choices.

Be mindful of your body:

Observe your body's feelings and reactions when following an endomorph diet. Monitor changes in appetite, feeling full, and overall well-being.

Speak With Experts:

See a physician, certified dietician, or personal trainer for guidance. They can give you sage advice and help you make educated decisions based on your achievements.

If you're not seeing the desired results, be open to making adjustments. This could mean altering the amount of food you consume, the way you exercise, or the ratios of nutrients in your food.

Appreciate Your Achievements:

Celebrate your successes, no matter how small. You can maintain your motivation and build healthy habits by appreciating and acknowledging your progress.

Regularly Reevaluate Your Goals:

Check your goals on a regular basis to make sure they still align with your goals and priorities.

Adjust goals as needed to keep yourself motivated and focused.

Possess endurance and patience:

Acknowledge that progress requires time. Keep up the steady work and be patient with the procedure. Success over the long haul demands constancy.

Remember that there is no one-size-fits-all endomorph diet or way of living. Individual responses vary, so you may need to make adjustments to the plan to make it meet your needs and preferences. Regular self-evaluation and professional guidance can help make an endomorph diet journey successful and long-lasting.

CONCLUSION

All things considered, the endomorph diet is a tailored approach designed to address the unique characteristics of individuals with an endomorphic body type, or those who tend to gain weight more easily. Partition control, a balanced intake of macronutrients, and a focus on nutrient-dense foods are the cornerstones of the endomorph diet. Regular exercise involving both aerobic and strength training is necessary to maintain a healthy weight and metabolism.

Individualization and adaptation are essential elements of the endomorph diet. By keeping a food journal, a fitness log, or regular evaluations, people can track their progress and gain more knowledge about how their bodies respond to dietary and lifestyle changes. It can also be quite helpful and encouraging to seek guidance from professionals such as certified dietitians, personal trainers, or medical specialists.

In the end, success on the endomorph diet requires tenacity, regularity, and a holistic approach to health. By practicing mindful eating, getting regular exercise, managing stress, and making adjustments based on individual reactions, people who identify as endomorphics can work towards achieving and maintaining their fitness and health goals in a sustainable way.

THE END